I0505517

CHART LIKE A PRO

New Nurses Charting Don't
Have To Be Complicated

YOUSELINE JEAN BAPTISTE

MERLANDE JEAN

Copyright © 2020

All rights reserved.

No part of this book may be used or reproduced by any means, graphic, electronic, or mechanical, including photocopying, recording, taping, or by any information storage retrieval system, without the written permission of the publisher except in the case of brief quotations embodied in critical articles and reviews.

Disclaimer

This book is only an informational guide from nurses to nurses. It's not a replacement of nursing laws or protocols but matter of fact encourages all nurse to follow nursing laws in there states and facilities.

Dedicated

This book is dedicated to all the new nurses. You are on the journey to caring for others health. May you become a beacon of hope and encouragement. May your work be filled with love and compassion for your patient. I hope that your work speaks for itself. May your passion always be the light that leads the way for you.

About the Authors

Youseline Jean Baptiste is an LPN for 10 years with experience and hospice, pediatric and drug detox and much more. She is the mother of three children also the CEO of Smart Nurse. She is a motivational speaker inspiring people to be great in everything they do.

Merlande Jean co-Author has been a nurse for over ten years. She started as an LPN and continue her education and become an RN. Her experience ranges from geriatric, urgent care and pediatric. Mother of two beautiful girls. Her goal is to continue growing in nursing and encouraging others to fulfill their dreams.

Table of Contents

Time, date, signature and error

In this chapter, you will learn about time, date, and signature, which is something you will always deal with. Your time and date need to be as accurate as possible. Try not to get in the habit of guessing your time. For example, you don't want to guess when you went to help a patient who fell, especially if you have a caregiver who has to write a report. Nurses and the patient care tech might often have conflicting times. It's okay to ask the caregiver what time they witnessed the incident instead of guessing. Your charting is a legal document, and if you understand that it is a legal document, then you know your time, date, and signature matters.

Let me explain. Mr. Street fell on your shift, and as of a result of the fall, he suffers several fractures and dies. The family decides to sue the facility, and now your notes are being reviewed by both lawyers.

Unfortunately, your notes can be used in a court of law by the other lawyer to prove neglect, medication error, and so forth. In this case, you wrote in your notes that the caregiver reported the patient fell at 8:20 pm, but the caregiver stated the patient fell at 8 pm, and she immediately reported it to the nurse, and that was you. But now there is a time discrepancy. A good lawyer will try to prove neglect, by asking, for example, why did you wait so long to attend to the patient after it was reported to you? Also, keep in mind that the EMS and the hospital also keep records with time such as when the patient came in, and the time the call was made to the EMS. So, if you think time does not matter, you are wrong.

Keynote: Avoid guessing your times.

Time overlap is a big issue. For example, you went to visit a patient, and, at your arrival, physical therapy is there or another healthcare worker. It is important that your visit time does not overlap with physical therapy or anyone else. When the company you work with tries to bill for these services, they usually can't get paid. Insurance companies see overlap as red flags for fraud, and this is a big deal in the healthcare industry. Unless you are told it is okay, always make sure when you are visiting a patient at their home for a nursing visit that it does not overlap other disciplines.

Keynote: Medicare charting can be very stringent.

With technology, you might have charting software where you can edit your time. The best way to make sure your time is accurate is to chart right away. Charting right away can be a challenge, so if you can't chart right away, write it down somewhere so you can get to the information when you need it. Never write on your hands. Believe me when I tell you nurses write things on their hands all the time and then wash their hands and only later when it's too late, do they remember they had something important written on their hands that they needed to chart. Nursing is a busy job, and you are going to have a lot of distractions. As soon as you think you are going to sit down to chart, an emergency happens, and you have to go see a patient, and that's when you wash your hands. So never chart on your hands.

Usually, your dates are fixed if you are using charting software, but if it's not just remember to include your date at the start of your note. Add the time with every new note entry. At the end of each note, make sure you include your signature. If you're still using pen and paper to chart, always use a black pen. If you make an error, make one straight line through it. Don't scribble. Sometimes you can write "error" right above the line. Figure out if there's a specific way your agency wants you to do it and go with that.

Protect any password concerning your charting login, etc. I repeat never give it out. But, if you must, change it immediately. You are responsible for your charting, not your boss or supervisor. Don't leave your password lying around, and don't leave your computer unattended. Even if you have to logout for a minute or two and log back in, which can be inconvenient, don't leave your computer screens open with patient information. This is not just for your protection. It is also for your patients' protection. It is part of your job to protect patient information. Make sure you understand the rules, and who to contact if you need to change your passcode.

Keynote: It is the law to protect your patient's medical record.

Priceless Advice Before Charting

Let's go over some very important things about charting that are priceless to your nursing career. This is where we talk about the importance of your nursing scope. So, what is the nursing scope?

The scope of practice describes the services that a nurse is qualified and competent to perform under the particular license they have. It is the law that governs the license you have.

This means if you are a Register Nurse or Licensed Practical Nurse, you will practice under the law that governs that license, and that includes your charting. Let's go over some examples.

Let's talk about certain things you should avoid doing.

The patient has a black, painful mole on the left cheek, which appears cancerous.

Even if you think it is cancerous, keep that to yourself. Sharing that information is not under your scope of practice. Do not diagnose patients or chart your opinion of the diagnosis, even if you are suggesting it might be cancerous or if you are stating it appears cancerous. Let the doctor make those types of calls. It's not part of the scope of nursing duties for an RN or LPN to diagnose.

Nurse completed head-to-toe assessment. Patient blood pressure is 165/72. Patient voices concern of high blood pressure. I stated to patient Hypertension was the cause of her high blood pressure.

What if you later found out that it was medication-induced and has nothing to do with him or her having hypertension? If you intend to keep your license, it is important to follow the law that governs that license. Don't be afraid of the law. Look at it as a protection. For example, if a patient pressured you for a diagnosis, you can honestly tell them you are waiting for the doctor to confirm that information, and at this point, you can neither confirm or deny whatever disease they think they have. The law protects you. The only time the law works against you is when you do things outside of your scope. If that patient reports you for not giving them a diagnosis, the law protects you. You don't have to operate out of your nursing scope because you are not a doctor. The only way the law works against you is when you're acting outside of your scope. Remember that.

Don't perform skills outside of nursing practice, which also means you shouldn't be charting outside of your scope. One of your jobs as a nurse is to know your nursing scope, which governs your license. So, you should never be charting skills outside of that license. It doesn't matter if you have the skills. If you receive your nursing education outside the U.S.A. and your skill is beyond what they teach here in America as a nurse, be careful to not use skills beyond your nursing scope or even think of charting skills outside of your nursing scope of practice. No matter how smart you feel or how much you want to impress a boss or co-worker, do not do it because you know how to do it, or you know how to do it safely. When it's out of your nursing scope, forget about it, or it raises a red flag. Don't charting outside of your nursing scope under any circumstance.

Keynote: Question you should ask yourself: Does your license or certification cover the skill you are performing or charting?

How about if you come from another state? Every state has its own rules and regulations. Or you are an independent contractor that works solo. The key thing is if you are in doubt whether you should perform a certain task or skill, find out. You can call the nursing board in whatever state you are in or go to their website.

Key: Remember, charting correctly is one thing, but charting under your nursing scope is a must.

Lastly, you must know the protocol for your nursing facility. Every hospital, nursing home, Assisted Living Facility, and home health has its protocol, and you should know the ones relating to you. When it comes to a medical facility, there's no one size fits all. You can't just operate under the last place you were working. Remember, every facility has its own protocol. Things might be slightly different, but that difference can be the difference between you making a phone call to the doctor or sending a patient to the hospital.

For example, you are charting about a patient's blood sugar results of 250. The protocol of some facilities might want you to notify the physician with that reading, but another facility might want you to notify the physician with a result of 300 or more. Understand that the slightest difference can matter. Some facilities might not have a sliding scale protocol for patients on insulin. Instead, it might just be patient specific. Your charting must be correct, but also in compliance with the protocol of the facility. It is part of your responsibility to know and follow the protocol.

Keynote: Every facility has its own policies and guidelines.

Objective and Subjective

As you continue to learn to chart correctly and accurately, you should know what objective and subjective data are and how to use them.

Objective

Any sign and symptom you can measure and observe.

Subjective

These are the patient experiences that you usually can't measure.

This is where you will hear what the patient states he or she is experiencing or feeling. What you need to remember is just because you can't prove what the patient states, never deny what the patient is saying he or she feels.

As you chart, always keep your feelings out of your charting. Your feeling is neither right nor wrong, but it definitely does not belong in your notes. If you feel like a patient is lying, your note is not the place for you to put things like I think the patient is lying. Never assume the patient is not telling the truth in your charting. Instead, chart exactly what the patient is doing so the reader can see your reasonable doubt. That way, you will not appear biased or discriminating. So leave your feelings out of your notes, and you will properly be able to deal with all patient concerns, whether they are subjective or objective.

Keynote: Show what a patient is doing rather than saying what you are feeling about what the patient is doing. Honestly, no one cares what you feel about the patient.

It's perfectly okay to chart what a patient states they feel. This is especially going to come into play when you are charting about pain. This where you will get a lot of subjective data and that information is going to be important when you have to give the patient an as-needed medication. When it comes to receiving subjective information from your patient, understand that they have the right to state what they feel even when you can't measure or observe what they are saying. Sometimes the only thing that's going to help justify you giving an as-needed pain medication or Ativan is that subjective data. Why else would you be giving an as needed Percocet 5mg when you just gave scheduled Tylenol 500mg or tramadol 50mg? You want to effectively note why you had to give an extra dose of pain medication.

Unfortunately, some nurses take the patient's narcotic medication for themselves. You never want to create unnecessary suspicion, so when you chart, it is necessary to put what the patient states they feel or experience. Because if anyone had to read your documentation to find out why the patient had to receive two extra doses of Percocet 5mg on your shift, even though you have an as-needed order, you might be the only nurse giving the as-needed medication. You have to CYA (Cover Your Ass). Make it clear why you gave the medication (Patient complaining of lower abdominal pain). It can also be that you've given the patient a scheduled Tylenol 500mg that was not effectively relieving the patient's pain. And you're going to give him his as-needed Tramadol 50mg. Don't forget to chart that subjective data—it should not be ignored. It should be clearly noted. It explains why you are giving that as-needed medication.

Here is one of the reasons subjective information should not be ignored. Say your patient complains to you about lower abdominal pain, and you document that information, but you fail to document your intervention. Then, something happens to that patient due to appendicitis, which caused abdominal pain, but you did nothing. You didn't even notify the physician or give pain medication. But you charted "patient complains of pain" without any intervention. This is not a good nursing judgment.

Let's look at another reason subjective data is important. When you document subjective data, it helps other nursing staff get a picture of the patient. When other medical staff, like physical therapy and so forth, read your charting, they might learn the patient may need pain medication before therapy and therefore ask the nurse on duty to give patient pain medication before physical therapy. Your charting also helps the nurse who needs to create a new care plan for the patient. So, understand that other staff members depend on your charting to get a clear picture of the patient's needs.

For example, a doctor may decide to increase pain medication or change the type of medication to something more effective. The doctor might notice every afternoon, his patient still complains of pain even after receiving the scheduled pain medication. I clearly understand doctors don't always read your documentation. The point to be taken is that subjective data not only helps you to better treat the patient, but the whole medical staff looking to care for that patient also benefits. If your documentation doesn't show that the patient is complaining of pain, then why are you giving that as-needed medication?

Do not look at your subjective data as useless information. It has its place and serves a purpose. Never ignore a patient's complaint because you believe they are an addict. That can very well be, but address that with the doctor or supervisor nurse. Never ignore their need and never chart your personal feelings about why you're not giving a patient pain medication. When you chart about not giving a patient medication, let it always be legal and follow protocol. Some orders might clearly state to hold medication if the patient is sedated. It has to be based on nursing judgment, not opinion. Don't document that you didn't feel the patient didn't need it, or the patient asked for too much medication. The bottom line is to keep your personal opinion to yourself. So, if you have to hold medication, make sure you are charting signs and symptoms if there are any, like drowsiness, lethargic, eyes are glazed over, gait is unstable and sedated. This will help you if you ever get a question as to why you didn't give the patient their pain medication. Your note will give a clear picture rather than just saying the patient didn't need more medication. Just in case a patient reports that you refused to give them their as-needed pain medication, you're covered.

Keynote: If you do not give a patient medication, make sure your reason follows doctor's orders, and it is in line with protocol. Never make it personal.

1/7/18 1530 Mr. Pathway receives Morphine 30mg by mouth as scheduled. Patient is alert to person, place, time, and event, and is watching tv and eating dinner. 1600 Patient requested as-needed morphine 15mg by mouth for breakthrough pain. Nurse assesses patient's eyes glazed over, slow movements, vital signs are within normal limits (blood pressure 128/75 Heart rate 82 Respiration 16 Temperature 97.5). Pain scale 5, patient complains of throbbing lower back pain. As-needed morphine 15mg (by mouth) for breakthrough pain held due to sign and symptoms of sedation. Nurse explains to patient he just received morphine 30mg 30 minutes ago when pain scale was 7. Patient encouraged to allow pain medication to work, which usually takes an hour. Nurse applies a heat pack to patient's lower back and repositions for comfort. Nurse asked patient did he have any questions about medication instructions. Patient stated he understands verbal instruction. Call light put in reach. Nurse will continue to monitor the effectiveness of medication and heating pack.

Don't forget to return to the patient to make sure what was implemented was effective and noted. Never forget to chart the outcome. Was it effective? If it wasn't, what did you do? If you don't do this part, why even bother charting the complaint? No one looking at your note will know it was effective. Final take away, there's a lot you could have added to the above charting, but the point is, are you listening and responding to patient needs? There is never a perfect way to work as a nurse or a perfect way to chart. But there are principles that you can apply to your work and your charting that will lead you to a more successful nursing career.

Abbreviation & Medical Terminology

Don't we love our abbreviations? But I have to tell you an important truth. During nursing school or in your nursing career, you are going to learn many abbreviations, and you have to be careful when using them. You can learn an abbreviation in one facility, but it might not be recognized in another facility. The last thing you want to happen is to use the abbreviation in your charting and have it confuse other nurses following behind your work. It can be an inconvenience to spell things out, and abbreviation can save time, but keep in the back of your mind that not everyone knows or uses the same abbreviation. If you cause confusion and there is a medical error due to your abbreviation, understand you are still liable. You will not be able to say I learned it in school. The facility can turn around and say we never approved that abbreviation, and you will be stuck.

Another thing you must take into consideration is that your charting can be view by many people and also some insurance companies who will be paying the hospital or medical facility for the care you perform. Different schools teach different abbreviations that might not be recognized across the board, but you should understand that nurses come from different schools and also different states and even other countries, and we don't learn the exact abbreviations. We might have the foundation of nursing skill, but abbreviations are not always common. I know not every facility is going to have approved abbreviations that nurses can use. Instead of taking a chance on an abbreviation you are unsure about, ask if the facility has an approved abbreviation list.

Keynote: Abbreviations are not always universally recognizable.

Medical terminology is one of the fun things we learn in school that makes us feel like a professional in the field, which basically means we speak the medical language, and that's awesome. But what we are not always aware of is our patients and their families usually don't speak medical terminology. Another thing that happens is we get so fluent speaking medical terminology we don't realize our patient is lost when we communicate to them and they might be too embarrassed to tell us. Medical terminology plays a role in our charting. I said this before, and I am going to say it again: your notes are legal documentation. Don't ever think they are exempt from the legal system. If something happens to a patient, their medical records will be one of the first things looked at. When it comes to medical terminology, it is important for you to know the definitions, your patient doesn't need to know it.

You should talk to the patient in layman's terms, and your charting should also reflect the real dialogue you had with the patient and not the medical terms. What you teach a patient, what you instruct a patient on, should be words they can understand, and when you chart that information, the person reading your notes needs to be clear that the instructions you gave your patient were understood without a doubt. This is also the reason why I haven't filled this book with a whole bunch of medical terminology and abbreviations.

Keynote: Medical terminology is for your understanding. Your patient needs to be talked to in a way they understand.

Assessment Charting

Assessment will always be a part of your nursing duties. Whether you are a Registered Nurse or Licensed Practical Nurse, you will chart about some type of assessment at least once during your shift. As a matter of fact, after receiving a report, you are probably going to start with assessing your patient. Remember, every assessment usually includes vital signs.

Let's start with patient alertness and orientation. If your patient is disorientated, confused, or unable to give consent, do not forget to include that throughout your charting. For example, Mrs. Planner is a 95-year-old patient with advanced Alzheimer's disease. You happen to give her medications, and if you charted she is not orientated to self, time, and place, you have to be careful that you do not chart things that contradict patient mental status, and if you do, you must clarify why. Did the patient's condition improve? Make it clear. In some circumstances, a patient might temporarily experience disorientation to self, person, and place, such as in the case of intoxication or when experiencing delirium.

Let's look at an assessment.

9/2/2000 0800 Mr. Hogue, a 97-year male patient is alert and oriented to person, place, time, and event sitting up in bed. No sign and symptoms of distress noted. Vital signs are within normal limits. Blood pressure 134/68. Heart rate 76, lung sounds are clear in all fields, respiration 18, and even, no respiratory distress noted. Patient denies chest pain. No signs and symptoms of infection noted, temperature 97.5. Bowel sound presents in all four quadrants, abdomen soft, and none tender. Last bowel movement 9/2/2000. BM formed, brown, medium. Patient voiding within normal limits, no s/s of infection. Patient denies urgency, frequency, and burning while urinating.

Patient c/o of muscle weakness ambulate with 1 person assist, patient is a fall risk, call light within reach, bed in a low position. Room and hallway are clutter-free to prevent falls. Skin intact, no open area noted. Pedal pause present and strong. Patient denies any pain or discomfort. Patient voices no concern to nursing at this time, will continue to monitor.

Now, the good thing is we have an evolving health industry. With technology, most companies are using electronic medical records making it so much easier to chart, because so much more could have gone into this one assessment. The software or assessment flow sheets make it easy not to miss things that can easily be overlooked. Most facilities use charting software, and within that software, there's an area for assessment. But don't allow technology to make you lazy or lose your critical thinking skills. Remember, charting software is always being improved on. It is not flawless. If there is not a place to add certain information about your assessment, do not ignore your findings. Get with a supervisor or nurse director to find a solution. Why? Because you are not going to be able to blame the software if you don't chart an important detail. Remember, your competency in passing the boards is why you hold your license. No type of charting software can take the place of that. The best way to chart assessment is to go from head to toes. But unfortunately, if you are writing your assessment, you might not get to write it or type it that way. What you must understand is that you need to include all the systems. Please understand that the software is there to help make things a bit easier and to improve documentation and record-keeping. Technology has also saved a lot of trees.

Keynote: When charting assessments, the best and most effective way to go from head to toes.

With every assessment, you have to address the chief complaint and get as much information regarding every patient complaint. Even if you were to do a head to toes assessment, it would not be thorough if it didn't assess the main reason the patient is in your facility. Remember, if a patient is in your facility ten-days, every day at the beginning of the shift patient should be assessed. Assessment is a huge part of a nurse's responsibility. Furthermore, how can you effectively take care of a patient if you don't know what's going on with that patient? Every time you start your shift, you're taking responsibility for every patient left in your care. Make yourself knowledgeable about those responsibilities. Never assume a patient's status will not change just because they were alert and orientated the day before. When it comes to assessment, one of the most important things to remember is to not forget to chart changes. Especially at the beginning of your shift, chart any finding that wasn't reported to you. I want you to understand there is a lot that goes into assessment, but we only touched on the basics since that is our focus in this book. You will continue to build on that foundation as you grow in your nursing career and build your skills.

Chart Admission & Discharge

In this chapter, here are the key things we will address since every facility has a different protocol. Let's go directly to some important things you might not realize. At the start of your admission, any wound or skin tear on the body should be noted. What usually happens if you don't chart these things is your facility owns the problem, which means your facility has to pay for it, and the problem could have started at another facility. So, if a patient walks in with any wound charted, for example, if your patient came from an assisted living to a skilled rehab where you work and the paperwork does not state the patient has a stage 2 skin breakdown, it is your job to chart that information if you are admitting that patient. At the time of admission, you have to properly chart patient condition. The last thing you want is your admission paperwork or computer charting to present your patient as someone who is in good condition when in reality, within a few hours, his or her condition might lead to the emergency room or ICU. That's why you can't just check off boxes. But don't just rely on the admission software or premade packages. Your admission is critical because you don't want all your charting to reflect healthy walkie talkie patients who then die at your facility. Be prepared within this time to note all subjective and objective data. Most charting software has a place to add additional information. To do admission properly, it takes experience, and that's not to discourage you, but for you to know the truth. If you are a brand-new nurse and you get thrown into the lion's den, or you took an admission job, it can be a challenge. Always ask for thorough training.

Some facilities have premade worksheets for admission and discharge if your facility has not started using technology. One of the biggest things concerning discharge you're going to have to fine-tune as a nurse is teaching your patient. No matter what premade worksheet or software your company invests in, it will not make you charting better. What it can do is make things easier, more organized, and help you not miss a step because the premade admission package and discharge worksheet tell you what to do next. A lot of nurses don't realize teaching patients and their families is a part of being a nurse, as well as being able to chart what was taught to the patient. Your discharge should not only complete the required form, but it should also give the patient clear instructions, and those instructions should be charted. Avoid a situation where someone says the nurse didn't tell me that, or she didn't say I have to take it twice a day. Also, this is the time you address any concerns a patient may have. Sometimes the reason why patients are readmitted after discharge is that instructions and teaching were not clear. Sometimes it takes a minute to ask a patient if they have any questions on a medication, especially if it a new medication or diagnosis. Ask them if they have any questions. Sometimes patients might not even know what question to ask, so go over as much as you can. Sometimes you don't even realize you might have answered a question for the patient. During the discharge process, it is really important that the patient leaves your facility with as much knowledge as possible about whom to call or follow up with. Unfortunately, a patient being readmitted is a huge concern for a lot of insurance providers. Discharge is not just getting the patient out of the facility. Sometimes patients don't understand what to do, or patients are confused and afraid of the diagnosis or bill, and they are not sure what to do next. It is our job as patient advocates to make sure we empower them with the information they need. Also, teaching is important because the insurance company wants to know exactly what you are instructing the patient on. And yes, they can deny payment or make it difficult if your charting does not show what you are doing for the patient. So, it is not just to make your charting look better than other nurses. With Medicare fraud and overpayment, these companies want to know the work is being done, and that includes the discharge, which is part of the teaching.

Keynote: Get comfortable teaching your patient.

How to chart refusals

What to do and not do

Don't just put down that the patient refused.

Patient refuses insulin.

Patient refuses care.

Patient refuses medication.

These are things nurses deal with daily. Let's go over some examples of charting refusals that are more effective. Also, keep in mind your writing style might be different from mine or another nurse, and that's okay. Good charting is painting a clear, concise picture of the problem and solution.

Patient refuses insulin. But what type of insulin? Did you notify anyone? What was the outcome? Did you teach the patient anything? The same thing goes for medications and refusal of care. What medication did the patient refuse? We, as nurses, are always charting. It's a big part of our job, and we can sometimes get lazy with it. I feel your pain; been there done that. But the more you get comfortable with charting correctly, the easier it gets.

Patient refused insulin.

1200 Patient blood Sugar is 145 and patient refuses Novolog 5 unit. Patient states she doesn't take insulin when blood sugar is 145 and she will not eat any bread. Nurse explained that bread was not the only factor in increasing blood sugar levels. Nurse went over the different things that contribute to high blood sugar. Instruction is given on Novolog injection and how it works to reduce high blood sugar. Patient was also instructed on how hyperglycemia (high blood sugar) affects the body. Patient has verbalized understanding of instruction and complication. Physician notified as ordered. Patient will continue to be monitored for signs and symptoms of hyper and hypoglycemia.

Patient refused AM blood pressure medication metoprolol 25mg. Blood pressure at 0800 138/72 patient stated she didn't feel it necessary to take metoprolol 25mg because her blood pressure was normal. Patient newly diagnosed with hypertension. This is the second refusal. Nurse instructed on hypertension and complication. Furthermore, education has been given on how metoprolol works. Nurse also allowed patient to ask any questions or voice concerns. Patient verbalized understanding of teaching and instructions. Patient insists she will only take medication if blood pressure is high. As protocol, MD notified. New order given to discontinue metoprolol 25mg tabs.

Remember, the patient has rights, and our job is not to infringe on those rights. The right to refuse care or medication is one of them, but you still have a job to educate and inform the patient.

Remember, you, as a nurse, are a problem solver. Don't chart a problem such as patient refused without intervention or implementation. Take every opportunity when a patient refuses to inform, to educate your patient on what's lacking in their understanding of the disease's process and medication. If you're ever in doubt, follow the protocol of your facility, use nursing judgment, and ask questions. God forbid the patient who refuses insulin experiences a complication and, as a result of hyperglycemia, is now in ICU. Family and doctor find out she didn't receive her noon or evening injection, and all you documented was the patient refused. Next thing you know, the family member is upset. The family members say she always refuses, and all you had to say is it was "sugar medication time and she would have received the shot."

Things that appear small might become bigger than life. The patient has the right to refuse, but don't just end it there. Remember, healthcare is a billion-dollar industry, and some people are looking for any opportunity to sue. Don't let your charting give them that opportunity.

Keynote: If you did not chart it, it was not done.

Charting Medication

The best way to chart about medication is by using the 8 Rights. It used to be 5 Rights, but in this book, we are going to focus on the 8 Rights.

Let's learn how to apply them.

Right Patient

Right Medication

Right Dose

Right Route

Right Frequency

Right Time

Right Site

Now, let's apply it to charting. Let's begin with the example of the Right Route. These are some of the mistakes I've seen nurses make, and I also have made some of these mistakes as well.

Patient took insulin or patient received insulin can both be incorrect and very confusing. What do you mean the patient took insulin? This doesn't answer the question of the Right Route, and that's what makes it incorrect. Took or receive doesn't tell us anything about the route because in nursing, it matters. As nurses, we should know a patient can be injured or even worse if a medication is given inaccurately. Charting what medication you gave is one thing, but how you gave it is another thing. Was it injected in the left arm, did the patient receive it orally, or did they receive it VIA peg-tube? You see, there are so many ways to give a medication. It's not enough to say a medication was received. Take the example of a medication given to a patient in the wrong route, and it injures that patient.

Let's take, for example, that you have a patient that claims you gave them their suppository Tylenol orally. Let's say that night when you gave the patient the suppository, the patient was a bit confused, but no one knows that also since there's no diagnosis at this time of confusion, and there has never been an issue with the patient remembering his or her medication. Instead of just your word against the patient's, your charting can help back up what you did and clear up the misunderstanding. Unfortunately, your notes did nothing to support what you said. Your charting reads:

2100 Patient received suppository Tylenol. Your charting did nothing to help you. Maybe the patient is right that he received the suppository Tylenol orally. No one knows where the patient received the suppository because your notes just stated the patient received it.

So, yes, use your 8 Rights, especially when charting about medication. You might not need to use all 8 but use them as a guide until you become comfortable.

Ask yourself is it received by mouth, which oral, is it sublingual, under the tongue, is it topical, on the skin. Keep all these things in mind when you chart for the first time. You might not think of these things. This is the process of thinking like a nurse, so enjoy doing it. Now let's look at the right dose. How many did the patient receive, two tablets, 10 units of Novolog? Using the 8 Rights helps you prevent medication errors, which is the purpose, but it can also be a guide to good charting. Your charting can be brief, but it must clearly show what was given and how it was given. When we do this, it eliminates speculation, and there's no need for guessing what you did or didn't do.

When you receive a verbal order, put in all the details of the 8 Rights. Doctors are human too, and they can leave out important information. So, if you are taking a verbal order, start using the 8 Rights as a guideline. Unfortunately, if you take an incomplete order from a doctor, you have to get in contact with that doctor and make that order correct.

Let's look at two orders, and you can tell me which ones are correct.

Ativan 10mg 1 tablet every night before bed for restlessness.

Tramadol 50mg 1 tablet by mouth for pain.

Did you figure it out? Well, neither one is correct. The first one is missing the Right Route. We don't know if it's by mouth or topical. Just because it says tablet, we shouldn't assume it's oral. It could be through a peg-tube. When it comes to medicine, guessing is dangerous.

Tramadol 50mg is missing frequency. How often does the patient get this medication? We know it is for treating pain, but we can't just give a patient pain medication whenever we want. Why? One big reason out of many is that the patient can overdose without a time frame. How would he or she know when they can take it again without a time frame? Or how long they should wait before taking medication again.

Nothing by Mouth

How about a patient that's NPO (Nothing by Mouth)? When charting NPO, you have to be careful because nurses often forget patients are NPO (nothing by mouth). Most of the time, a patient becomes NPO due to a procedure they are going to have some time after a procedure. So be clear when you are charting to follow the doctor's order. If the doctor states nothing by mouth after 12 am blood pressure medication metropole 25mg only with ice chip. Please make sure you not only follow those orders, but you clearly chart what you did according to orders. Sometimes patients are permanently NPO if they have a peg-tube. The last thing you want to do is chart that you are given oral medication to a patient who just became NPO or has NPO. That's why it is important to keep the 8 Rights of medication. Your chart needs to reflect that because it's a medication error to give patient medication in the wrong route. So, pay attention to effectively caring for the patient and correctly charting your work.

Dealing with Medication Error

Okay, so what happens if you accidentally give oral medication to a patient who is nothing by mouth. The first thing I hope is that you catch yourself and use proper nursing judgment and protocol to ensure patient safety. What I can say is, never ignore a mistake you've made. Unfortunately, medication error does happen, even to the best nurses. In those instances, assuring patient recovery and safety is always placed first before charting. After that, you chart the event that occurred. You will probably write an incident report for the facility that is usually not put with the chart. After you clearly state what occurred, make sure you clearly state the outcome. The outcome is going to be vital just in case there's a lawsuit later.

It's always scary when something unintended occurs, but every great business understands it is inevitable. No matter how great the company or nurse is, things happen. So, breathe, use nursing judgment, and follow protocol. Patient safety and outcome is really important after the incident. Chart if the patient is now laughing and all vital signs are within normal limits. Make it clear. If you called the doctor, make note of the call and the order given. Was the patient sent to the hospital? What action did you take? Remember, if there is a lawsuit, your charting can be what saves you or crucifies you. The representative attorney is going to go through your charting with a fine-tooth comb. It might be something simple you missed, or no charting was done till the next shift. So, follow protocol. Some facilities want you to chart on patients every two hours or every hour. That's where your nursing judgment comes in. Even though you've charted a thorough note about the event and outcome, go back and check-up. Have a patient care tech do check-ups on the patient and follow up with you regarding the patient. Never assume the next nurse is going to pick up where you left off at the end of your shift. Thoroughly document patient activity, mental status, vital signs, and the condition you are leaving the patient in. This is important because nothing can fall back on you. You do not want your charting to appear like you neglected your patient, especially after an incident. You can't blame a patient lawyer for making you look incompetent or negligent. They are doing their job. Cover yourself and make sure your patient care is charted thoroughly under these events and circumstances.

Charting Coworker's Names

When charting, be very careful using staff names. Your charting is not a place for a smear campaign if you don't like the caregiver or your supervisor, and you don't feel like they are doing their job. Charting something like, "I told Lee Moore all afternoon to check up on Mr. Broom. Patient fell out of bed." That's a big red flag for a lawsuit. Let me make it clear that the patient or the patient's family has the right to sue if their loved one has an injury due to neglect and so forth. With that said, your job is not about making it easier to get your facility sued. You can talk to a supervisor on duty if you have a problem with a co-worker. But if you must write or type one of your colleague names, make sure you are professional and keep your disagreement or dislike out of your charting.

Charting Pain

When it comes to pain, there are some important basic questions you must ask your patient to effectively treat their pain and to chart properly. Let's get right into it.

Know where the patient's pain is and what the pain is doing. Is the pain radiating anywhere? Is it a constant pain or intermittent pain? Is the pain only with movement? Once you know the movement of the pain, you want to know the type of pain it is. Sharp, dull, or throbbing. When did this pain start? Is it acute or chronic?

You're going to need to know the pain scale and what makes it worse or better.

Location: Abdomen, leg, hip.

Provoking factors: Such as, when patient eats pizza, patient experiences upset stomach.

Pain type: Sharp, throbbing, burning, stabbing, do pain radiate anywhere.

Pain scale: On a scale 1 through 10.

Onset: Acute or Chronic.

What makes it better or worse: Movement makes it worse. When patient rests, pain subsides.

A lot of times, your patient is not going to be able to tell you they are experiencing pain. So how do you know the proper way to chart that?

Nurse completed 0900 assessment, patient up in chair grimacing and sobbing after being repositioned from bed to chair. 0910 Nurse gave patient tramadol 50mg tab PRN by mouth for pain. 1010 patient reassessed for pain. No s/s of distress noted patient is pleasant and comfortable eating toast and scrambled eggs. Patient continues to be monitored for comfort and safety measures.

2/5/19 1655 Patient reported tightness and pressure around her forehead, pain scale of 6. Patient states movement makes pain worsen and is experiencing headache for 17 years when in stress. 1715 Patient was given Tylenol 500mg one tab by mouth per physician order. 1815 patient reevaluated, patient in bed, resting comfortably watching tv. Patient denies pain and discomfort, states pain scale of 0.

Remember, there are a lot of other things that can be added to the above note. Our focus being pain, but we could have added patient mental status or vital signs. You are always going to use your nursing judgment at all times. Not only when you are caring for the patient, but also with your charting. Once all is done, your chart will be what reflects your work.

Key: One of the important keys when charting about pain is reevaluating the effectiveness of the medication. Don't forget that step. Try not to skip it.

Just because you state you gave a patient pain medication, does not mean everything is okay. A patient can turn around and state they were in pain all night, and if the last thing you charted was you gave tramadol 50mg and you never went back to make sure the medication was effective, that needs to be charted as well.

Antibiotics

First, I am going to start off by saying some facilities have a specific protocol they want you to follow while your patient is on an antibiotic. There are a few instances where patients are on antibiotics for life, but most of the time, this is not the case. With antibiotics, we are dealing with some type of infection, and infection control is a big deal. As a nurse, we always want to limit the spread of any infection. So, when a patient gets a urinary tract infection or upper respiratory infection, our goal is not only to get our patient infection free but also to stop the spread of infection, which often can be neglected. Imagine a case with one patient with C-difficile and then ending up with four to six patients with C-diff that they got while in your facility. So, it is very important to not only treat patients per MD orders but also to use infection control protocol. That means when you are charting, don't just chart your usual practice but also add your prevention. This does not have to be long and drawn out, but your prevention measure must not only be in place and implemented but charted as well.

Say there was an outbreak of some kind and the health department and other agencies came to your building and looked at medical records. And all your charting is great except there is no real evidence that the staff used infection control measures. Now the agencies want to do a full-blown investigation. Unfortunately, in the health care field, medical staff is sometimes the biggest contributor to passing on the infection. Everyone knows nurses are taking care of multiple patients. One of the biggest infection preventions is handwashing. When we chart, we are not just showing what we are doing for the infection, but we should also show what we are doing to prevent and protect the patient from getting an infection. Okay, it is your job as a nurse to know signs and symptoms of infection.

There are classic things we are going to look for with any infection. Monitor temperature. Abnormal temperature and fever can be an indicator of infection. Vomiting, redness, and pus can vary depending on the type or location of infection. Sometimes patients may be asymptomatic, which means they have no signs or symptoms, but it doesn't mean they don't have an infection.

Key point: If you have to call a doctor for a patient, most likely, you're going to receive a medication order. Always be aware of any allergy that the patient may have.

2/24/16 0800 Mrs. Bigbear states she doesn't feel like herself. Patient refuses to go down for breakfast. Breakfast brought up to patient's room. Patient is encouraged to eat and drink. The patient received her favorite breakfast of scrambled eggs and toast. When the nurse asks is there something else she can get the patient, the patient stated no, I am not feeling well today. Nurse assessment completed patient alert and oriented to person, time, place, and event, patient blood pressure 128/76 heart rate. 101 resp 18 even. Patient denies chest pain, no sign and symptom of distress. The temperature is 102. Patient complains of abdominal pain and tenderness, mild distention noted. Nurse verified bowel movement noted in flow sheet, patient had a medium, soft bowel movement at 0700. Patient skin is dry. 0810 nurse notified physician on-call order receive for Tylenol 500mg one tab every six hours by mouth for pain and fever. Uranalysis culture and sensitivity stat ordered. Verbal order read back.

Your personal charting style has nothing to do with charting effectively. For example, I have seen different ways nurse chart things. What's going to be important is that you convey a clear picture. If your boss or I was reading your charting, would I know the exact problem and how you, as a nurse, have been solving or treating your patient's problem? If you have clearly shown the problem and what you are implementing and identified the outcome of that implementation, you are on your way to charting like a pro.

Outcomes

We've spoken so much about outcome that it is only fair to dedicate a chapter to the subject. By now, you should already have learned outcome is a big part of your charting. It is what makes your notes complete. The outcome is the result of all your hard work. Without it, nobody knows what really happened. You might not be noting a result for every note you complete. But let's look at an instance where it's a must.

You got a stat order to give Mr. Clover Clonidine 20mg because when you took his vital sign this morning, his blood pressure was 185/114. After giving the Clonidine, would I go back after an hour, recheck the blood pressure and document the new result? I would. You are asking for trouble if you just give the medication and don't follow up. A clear picture means you charted a patient's high blood pressure, which you had to call the physician about. The doctor gives you a one-time stat order. You give the patient the medication, but your charting doesn't stop there. You have to add the outcome to have a complete note. Also, if the outcome was blood pressure is still very high, your charting is not done, and this is the phase where you need to be using nursing judgment. Remember, until the issue is resolved, your charting is not complete. Imagine you've thoroughly charted about a patient's condition or you've charted about something you implemented, but you never told us what happened after you implemented such and such. No one knows what happens, so any time you leave out your outcome, your charting is incomplete.

The problem is the reason for your care. The chief complaint is your WHY. Implementation is the order in which you execute the things you must do. What are you going to do for your patient?

Outcome was the result of what you did. Was it effective? Do we need to continue monitoring? Are we progressing with the care of plan? Do we need to call the doctor because the medication is not effective?

PROBLEM

IMPLEMENTATION

OUTCOME

Let's look at some examples

4/3/2015 0900 patient received the last dose of ciprofloxacin 500mg by mouth tablet. Vital signs within normal limits. Heart rate 86 Blood pressure 122/65 Respiration is Even 18, no sign and symptom of distress, temp 98.5. Patient denies pain and discomfort. Nursing instruction given patient will stay hydrated throughout the day. Patient states she understands she must avoid dehydration, which can cause UTI. Patient states she is following physician's order drinking plenty of water throughout the day. Nurse reviews the signs and symptoms of dehydration. Some of the symptoms are thirst, dry or sticky mouth, dark yellow pee (urine) patient has verbalized understanding of the symptoms. The patient states she is urinating pale yellow pee, no distention noted of the abdomen, denies urgency, burning, and frequency while peeing (urinating.) No signs and symptoms of infection noted. Patient also states she is drinking four cups to five cups of water a day.

So, you're not just giving ciprofloxacin 500mg, you are giving a complete picture to indicate the infection is resolved and the patient is free of the signs and symptoms of infection.

Keynote: You must document your outcome, which is your result.

Sometimes a patient can have a chronic disease where a lot of what you are doing is management care or preventative care. For example, with preventive care, you might be given medication to prevent myocardial infarction, and you might think you don't have any results to document and all you have to do is give this medication. But throughout your shift, or when you are doing your last notes on that patient, you chart that the patient is in stable condition and the vital signs are within normal limits. That is the patient outcome. Don't think there isn't an outcome. As a result of you executing a doctor's order and giving great patient care, your patient remains stable and free of nosocomial infection and safe throughout your shift. As nurses, we do not realize how much we do and how all that plays into the patient outcome.

Keynote: Remember, everything you are doing is playing into your patient's outcome. That also includes everything you should have done that you didn't.

The Three-Phases of Looking at Charting

PROBLEM

INTERVENTION /IMPLEMENTATION

OUTCOME

Putting It All Together

Your problem: Is the reason why.

Your intervention OR implementation is your action.

Your outcome: is your result.

Phase 1: Let's start with the problem: The first step is the reason we are caring for the patient. What is the reason you are given antibiotic medication?

Phase 2: Your intervention or implementation, which will be your action, will be based on your phase

1 patient need, which is the reason they are here.

Phase 3: The outcome of the thing you implemented. The outcome of the pain medication. Outcome of a wound that needs to be measured weekly. An outcome of a patient who fell.

Do not Give Up

Charting will be a big part of your job, and as nurses, most schools barely go over charting. Some brush over it lightly, some give it no attention at all.

You can't do anything effectively with a negative attitude. Instead of letting fear control you, understand you are not in this alone. Start creating a positive mindset that you can chart effectively. What you believe you can do, you will do.

Have goals when you start your nursing career about what you want to achieve by year one, year two, and year three. Let good charting be one of them.

Believe that the facility where you work wants you to win because it costs money to hire and train, so start working with having a positive mindset. People believe in you, and they are rooting for your success.

Never be afraid to ask for help. Remember, there's always someone willing to help you.

Never give up if at first you don't succeed. Be willing to keep putting out the effort. Charting is a skill, and you will eventually learn and even go beyond this book. So, give yourself a break, and don't give up on your career.

Final word

I didn't fill this book full of examples for good reason. First, that was not my goal. Secondly, I hope you get the point that you're going to have to use your judgment and that there are no perfect templates. Be prepared to change with technology because it is going to completely revolutionize how we chart and take care of our patients. Remember, every patient is unique. You will not be able to copy your way in nursing. Nursing requires judgment, and you will not be able to get away from that. That is one of the reasons you got the license. You passed boards and showed competency. Now use it. Every diagnosis is going to be unique to that patient. You don't have to be perfect, but you must clearly show your work with your charting. Nothing in this book is going to be able to replace your nursing judgment or the law that governs your license or the protocol of the facility where you work. This book is about empowering you to give you some starter knowledge from nurse to nurse. But remember, receiving that license means you are held to high regard. I want you to know I believe in you. I understand your struggles. I want you to know it can be scary at first, and if you have been at this for some time, remember that things will get better. You just have to be willing to put in some work and effort. Nursing is a demanding field, and there's room for every nurse to be successful. I wish you the very best on your nursing journey.

www.ingramcontent.com/pod-product-compliance
Lightning Source LLC
Chambersburg PA
CBHW021503210526

45463CB00002B/868